YOUR BREATHING

COACH

JULIA RUDAKOVA

You are here not to reach
the final healing point -
that is an illusion.

You are here to walk the
path, learn and get better
along the way,
to be able to say one day:
"I brought some joy
into this world,
and that's enough."

TABLE OF CONTENTS

INTRODUCTION

I was born in cold, central Russia, where the lowest winter temperature I remember from my childhood was something around -40° (that's 40 degrees below zero). It got real. If you think you can mouth breathe in those conditions, you are wrong. Culturally it was also emphasised to children, from a very young age, that it wasn't ok to breathe through the mouth as it was perceived as impolite behaviour. "Close your mouth", "chew with your mouth closed" – those phrases were used by parents a lot. In the English language the term "mouth breather" has a definition in the dictionary of "a stupid person". It comes from the fact that mouth breathing actually changes the shape of the cranio-facial bones, neck posture and makes people look less attractive, speaking statistically.

Interestingly, despite the fact that it was stemming from climatic and cultural circumstances and that parents were unaware of the importance of nasal breathing on the physiological level and how it affects the whole chemistry in the body, that particular aspect of parenting worked regardless of the reasoning behind it.

I thought I'd mention this as it used to be common to breathe through the nose just a few decades ago, while nowadays mouth breathing is normalised by the medical industry. You can hear "the child may grow out of it" or "we will take the tonsils out; he will breathe better again" or no comments AT ALL at general practitioner or maternal and child health nurse appointments. With advances in the pharmaceutical industry, it is more acceptable to medicate blocked noses, cut out tissues that interfere with nasal breathing and do absolutely nothing to address the root cause of why nasal breathing became difficult in the first place. None of the conventional therapies, which are used for congestive, upper-respiratory tract issues, work long term or resolve them.

It is a combination of lifestyle changes (nutrition, gut health), retraining the brain and the body to breathe better (consider it a gym for the brain) and, if need be, doing some mindset/ emotional work to address why the body is sending these signals about the most vital function of the body – breathing.

The WHY of breathwork

1. Internal body chemistry: via breath we oxygenate (= provide energy) to all cells and tissues in the body; influence our pH (acid-base balance); support blood glucose metabolism; maintain healthy oxygen-to-carbon dioxide ratio (meaning keeping the muscles happy, cells oxygenated).

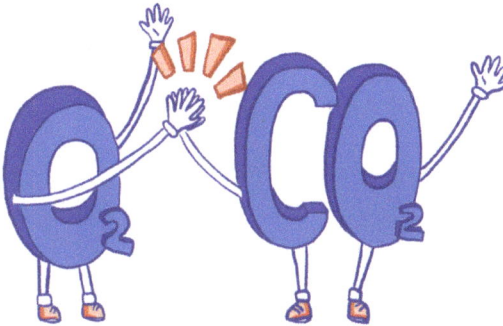

2. Mind: with the correct breathing mechanics, you calm the mind via down regulating the stress response. This is achieved through both the vagus nerve stimulation when engaging the primary breathing muscles and using an acupressure point in the middle of the roof of the mouth, slowing the heart rate and reducing anxiety. The latter is achieved by the tongue naturally pressing on the roof of the mouth when the mouth is closed. This connects two main meridians (also known as energy channels in

the body, according to Traditional Chinese Medicine), which brings calmness, increases stamina and gives more connection to the internal forces of the body.

3. Soul: the word "respiration" has "spirit" as its root; all spiritual practices have various breathwork types as an important part of them, even when we look at mantras used in Buddhist and Hindu religions, their rhythm and length are coordinated with the breath.

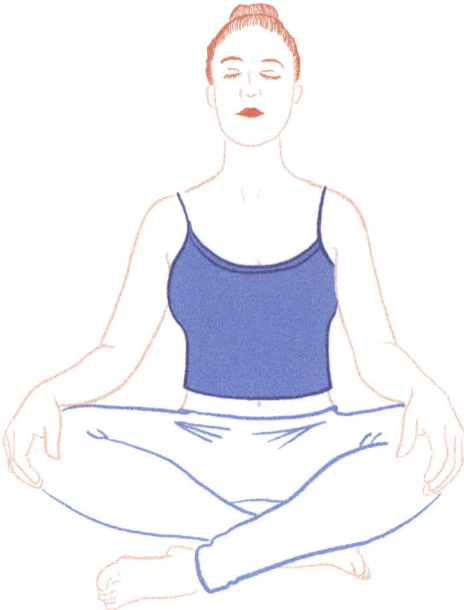

4. Intuition: breathwork allows you to deepen your intuition by bringing you fully into the body, using the diaphragm and activating the solar plexus energy centre, your gut centre. You connect that with your heart (through the rhythmical breath) and head as the diaphragm muscle is innervated by the phrenic nerve. Curiously, the Greek term "phren" means "mind" or "diaphragm" and up until the 19th century it was thought that the mind sits in the diaphragm.

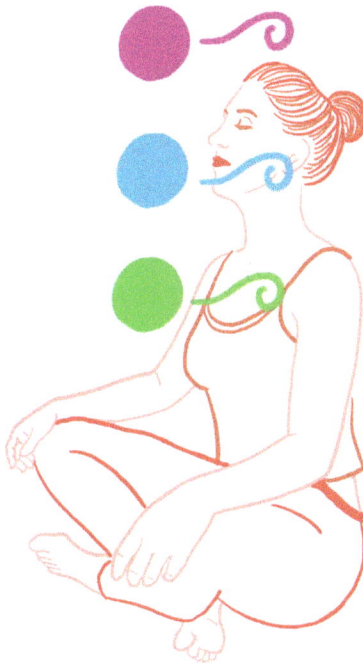

5. Breathing is the best, cheapest (well, actually, completely free!), most easily accessible medicine, which is always at your disposal, always at your command.

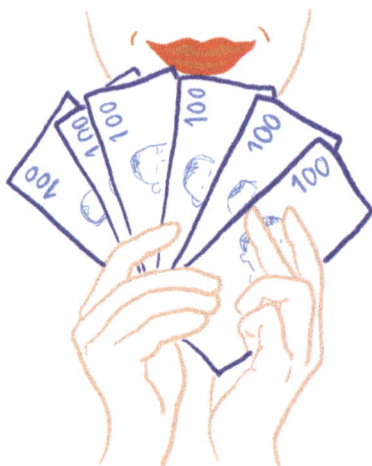

What is functional breathing?

Functional in this context means optimal; it means that all systems in the body work in an optimal way, providing you with energy for your inspired daily actions.

Functional breathing techniques will help correct the biochemistry in the blood, allowing for better oxygenation of cells and, as a result, better focus and concentration and increased energy levels, as oxygen is a source of energy. Functional breathing ensures optimised recovery after physical exertion, less lactic acid build up and improved stamina.

Functional breathing improves digestion and the assimilation of nutrients, plays a significant role in getting a better-quality sleep, deeper relaxation and promotes more vitality in general.

This book is your personal breathing coach, which provides you with comprehensive and concise information and step-by step instructions on how to retrain your body to breathe for optimal health.

I have been researching and practicing breathwork for over 25 years now, so I am able to put all the knowledge I accumulated in a practical, no-fluff form so that you get all the crucial information and exercises in a concise version, and you can start practising today. If you read only 2-3 pages a day, you will be a decent breathwork specialist within a month and will be able to maintain the routine and results as your lifestyle choice and enjoy good health. Remember, that breathing is the first medicine, which comes even before nutrition.

"If you feel that you have made a mistake, you don't try to undo the past or the present, but you just accept where you are and work from there."

Chögyam Trungpa

BALANCE AND CORRECT

The goal of this chapter is to bring your awareness to your breathing pattern. To get you to where you want to be in your health, you must establish where you are now as honestly and objectively as possible. The way you breathe can tell you a lot about the state of your health. This chapter is also about balancing, bringing your body to the point of neutrality, so that you can safely build up from that.

Breathing for balancing the nervous system

No matter what you are seeking – more energy or easier and deeper relaxation – you have got to calm and balance your nervous system first. The nervous system governs your respiration, rules your breathing pattern. But the good news is that it is a two-way street and, by controlling your breath, you can affect your nervous system as well. And this is exactly what we are going to do.

Your nervous system has two branches – sympathetic and parasympathetic nervous systems.

Sympathetic nervous system is also called "fight or flight" or stress response. It is the system that is activated when the body experiences a perceived danger or an expectation of the unknown. In the past, most dangers were real – running away from a predator was one of the common ones. Nowadays, it is more about perceived stress, rather than real physical danger. For example, there was a study that showed that even before opening an email, our stress hormones level go up. A modern person deals with psychological stress of relationships at work and home, finances, driving, as well as chemical stressors (toxins in food, environment, etc.). In short, you may have a lot of sympathetic nervous system triggers, which brings you to, what is called, sympathetic nervous system dominance.

Parasympathetic nervous system is your "rest and digest" system. The signs of being in the parasympathetic mode are slower heart rate, relaxed muscles, reduced body activity (as opposed to the sympathetic mode, when the body is ready to act and is in an alert state to fight or run for your life). Examples of parasympathetic nervous system states are sleep, meditation, digesting following a meal, the calm you experience when out in nature.

This chapter is about HOW to balance those two nervous system branches and take you out of the sympathetic nervous system dominance. When parasympathetic ("rest and digest") nervous system is upregulated (meaning – balances out the "fight or flight" response), then, and only then, can you say that your breathing pattern is functional – your organs are working at their optimal level, all tissues are receiving the right amount of oxygen, your muscles recover well after physical exercise. A well-regulated nervous system means great overall health.

As mentioned previously, our breathing is automatic. We don't have to think about how to breathe, and our breath is influenced by our nervous system. However, we can also DIRECT our breath, consciously affecting our breathing pattern. If you have a poor tolerance of carbon dioxide (in functional breathing retraining we use a "control pause" test to figure out your CO_2 tolerance level), you may experience some challenges when doing the exercises outlined here. The reward of more energy, better sleep, and improved mood is so worth it!

Take time to go through the following steps as this is **the foundation of functional breathing**. I recommend to focus on one principle a day and practice it with commitment and focus.

Correcting your breathing pattern starts with awareness

Become aware of the way you breathe. While sitting with this book in front of you, start observing the following:

Your breathing pattern checklist

Do you breathe through the nose or mouth most often?

Notice if there are dribbles on the pillow case in the morning, if your lips are dry, if your lips are slightly apart when working, driving or watching TV.

Do you breathe with the chest or abdomen?

What is moving when you breathe? Is it chest, shoulders, belly?

Do you breathe fast or slowly?

Open the Stopwatch app on your phone and time how many breaths per minute you take.
One breath = inhalation + exhalation.
If you score below 8 - fantastic! If your score is more than 8 breaths per minute, you will be able to reduce your breathing rate with the help of the exercises in the book.

Do you breathe loudly or quietly?

Start to take note of other people's breathing when you sit next to them at the table or in public transport. If you can't notice how audible your breathing is, ask a friend if they can hear you breathe when you are in close proximity and don't talk to each other.

All the activities above are to be done without judgement, just as an observation.

Correcting your breathing pattern

Nasal breathing

First, you absolutely must re-establish **nasal breathing**.

Here's a visual for you. Remember, as a child, you were lying on the floor or a couch, watching dust particles dancing in the sunrays? Outdoors the tiny air-borne particle storm is even denser – pollens, dusts, diesel fuel exhausts, etc. The nose is our advanced technology of air-conditioning, which lungs can't do without. Our lungs love filtered, moist, warm air, and that's exactly what the nose does – filters, warms, and moistens the air for the lungs. When using the mouth to breathe, you bypass that filtration and conditioning system, and the lungs receive dry, cold and unfiltered air. When air of that quality enters the lungs, the bronchi will start to produce mucus to expel the dust and to moisten the environment. How does that manifest? A person will develop coughs and excess phlegm. Another important aspect of nasal breathing is that we produce nitric oxide in the nasal cavity, and it is our first line of defence against microbes, as it has an anti-microbial action; nitric oxide also plays an important role in vasoregulation – the opening and closing of blood vessels; helps to keep arteries young and flexible; participates in neurotransmission; helps regulate blood pressure. The latter is one of the most prominent functions of nitric oxide (NO) - its action on the arteries and blood pressure regulation. Because of that NO is known as a preventer of strokes, heart attacks, and other cardio-vascular symptoms.

Doctor Buteyko, the founder of the breathing method with

his name, cured his severe hypertension by practicing what he preached – slow nasal diaphragmatic breathing. He also developed a series of exercises, used in this book, to further improve cardio-vascular function.

"Nasal breathing ensures the perfect chemistry in the body and minimises respiratory distress."

Important!

The only contraindication to the exercises is severe obstruction in the nasal cavity (very large adenoids in children or extremely deviated septum in either children or adults). How do we check? Make sure the mouth is closed, lips together and set the timer for one minute. If you can breathe through your nose for at least one minute, breathing retraining is possible, you may proceed with the functional breathing exercises and start implementing the basic principles of functional breathing.

Breathing mechanics

This is the most overlooked aspect of breathwork. The best I heard was "breathe into the tummy", which is not a bad start. However, there are a lot of misconceptions about tummy breathing versus chest breathing. It is a little more complicated than that. We are not dissimilar to other mammals, in terms of the mechanics of breathing. We primarily use the diaphragm and intercostal muscles (the ones between your ribs) to breathe. The abdomen moves slightly, but abdominal muscles are not the breathing muscles, they do not drive the process of respiration.

Two most common mechanical faults I see in my clients are inverted breathing (when the abdomen deflates upon inhalation and balloons out when exhaling) and engaging chest muscles for breathing instead of relying on the diaphragm and intercostals. The intercostal muscles tend to get lazy overtime if not used regularly. "Use it or lose it" is applicable to any bodily function!

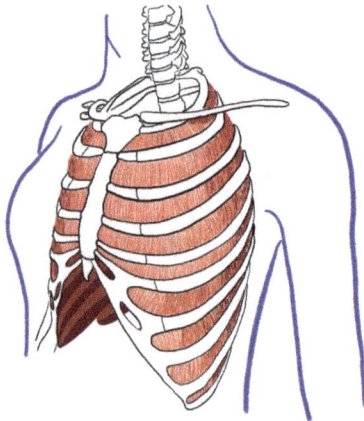

Correction exercises

In "Your breathing pattern checklist" section on page 18, you have gone through the main points of functional breathing. Now that you have noticed what you're doing mechanically when you breathe, it's time to correct (or reinforce, in case you're engaging all the right breathing muscles) your breathing mechanics.

Correction exercise 1

Focus on your lower ribs, put your palms on the sides of your lower rib cage and expand them laterally (push into your hands) as you breathe in and contract (allow your hands to come closer) as you breathe out. You can use a resistance rubber band to strengthen the lateral/horizontal breathing pattern.

How to:

Wrap your resistance band around the lower ribs, hold the ends, crossed, in front of you. Breathe for 2-3 minutes - slowly, through the nose, feeling the resistance of the band when you inhale. Incorporate this exercise during your breaks at work. This exercise helps the intercostal muscles and the diaphragm.

To really appreciate your intercostal muscles and feel them at work, push your thumb between your two lower ribs and notice how your thumb sinks in between the ribs as they come apart on the inhale and then come together on the exhale, pushing the thumb out.

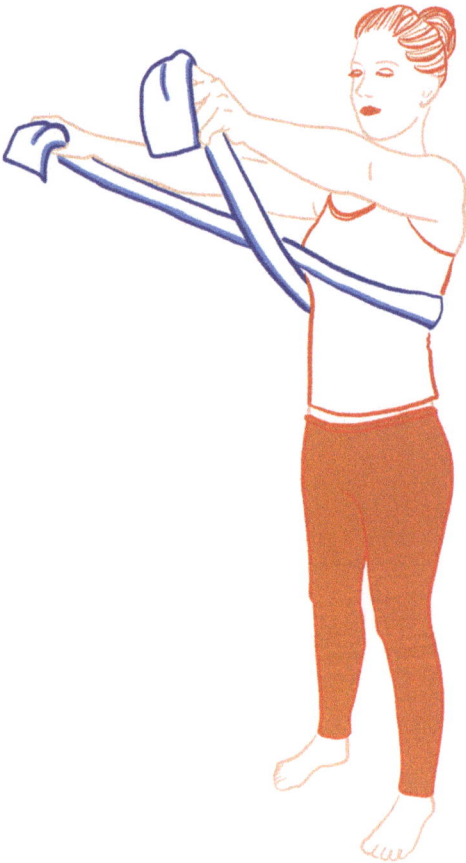

Correction exercise 2

Another way of starting to get the right diaphragmatic action is to lie on a firm, flat surface (yoga mat/rug on the floor), knees bent. Put a heavy book on your belly and breathe slowly - breathe in to the count of 4, breathe out to the count of 6. You are going to move your book up on inhalation and down on exhalation. Do not worry if the count 4 and 6 is stressful. At the initial stage some people find it hard to slow down their breath. Experiment! Try 3 and 5 or 2 and 4. The only requirement is that your exhalation is longer than inhalation. The reason for that is that the sympathetic nervous system drives your inhalation, and the parasympathetic nervous system is responsible for exhalation. Functionally, our breath out is longer than the breath in when the parasympathetic ("rest and digest") system is balanced.

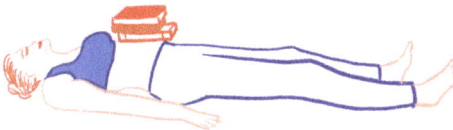

Inhale

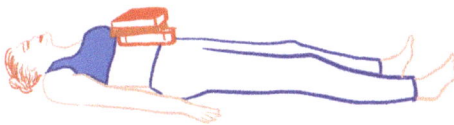

Exhale

"Learn how to exhale, the inhale will take care of itself."

Carla Melucci Ardito

What I have been observing in the clinic is that it is challenging for most clients who start the Functional Breathing Program with me, to exhale longer than to inhale. Have a stopwatch on your phone handy and time your breathing rate and the length of your exhalations. See if they are equal to, shorter or longer than your inhalations.

Your task here is to focus on consciously changing the pattern of shorter exhalation to lay the foundation for good health.

Once you have mastered 4:6 breathing and the book on your stomach, which you're using for training, is moving up and down with your in and out breath, put your hands on the sides of your lower ribs and imagine them pushing into your palms when inhaling. Now, press the ribs together when exhaling, imagining your waist going small. You can also feel your spine pushing into the mat slightly, ensuring a 360-degree breathing pattern.

Practice this:

SLOW (4:6)

GENTLE

(no sound coming in and out of your nostrils when you breathe – "breathe as if you are not breathing")

NASAL

DIAPHRAGMATIC

breathing daily, for at least 15 minutes.

It is a fantastic way of winding down after a work/school day.

To sum up, there are TWO aspects in the "Focus and Correct" stage of breathing retraining: **nasal**, gentle, inaudible breathing AND diaphragmatic, 360-degree **breathing mechanics**.

"Every action you take is a vote for the person you wish to become."

James Clear

OPTIMISE AND ENHANCE

This chapter is all about practice. At the initial stages of breathing retraining I recommend making time for regular practice AND weaving mini-practices throughout the day.

By the end of this chapter, if you are consistent with your daily practice, you will have greatly improved your tolerance to carbon dioxide, which is important for stamina, better recovery after any physical training or exercise, increased oxygenation of the cells and tissues, reduction of respiratory symptoms and optimal pH in the body.

Checklist

You will need:

1. Stopwatch and timer on your phone or a separate gadget;
2. Resistance rubber band (or a scarf/belt);
3. Mouth tape (any type – Myotape and Micropore tape are the two varieties I use in my clinical practice with both children and adults);
4. Nasal dilators, if necessary (I am not going into depth about them here, but if you used them in the past, you could experiment with them while doing your breathing retraining);
5. A burning desire to live a healthier life.

Keen to see your true level of fitness and how effectively your body utilises oxygen? Here is a very specific activity for that. This exercise also serves as a tool to measure your progress in the functional breathing work.

As breathing is an extremely subjective process (we all add our judgement to how we breathe – the pace, depth, etc.), it is a good idea to have some sort of metric to track your progress. I encourage you to measure your control pause (CP) every morning upon waking. That's right – when you put your feet down on the floor while sitting on your bed, grab a stopwatch and do your CP measurement. To do this, wait until you naturally EXHALE, pinch your nose (you MUST block your nostrils for this measurement as air is gas, and we must ensure a clear experiment), start the stopwatch and hold your breath until the first urge to breathe. DO NOT hold your breath as a competition! This is a

COMFORTABLE breath hold, which means, that when you release the hold, you should be able to continue breathing normally through the NOSE without signs of distress (for example, after a competitive breath hold, upon release of the hold, you would experience a big, very audible inhalation, which is a sign of respiratory distress). After the comfortable breath hold in the CP, your inhalation upon the release of the hold should not be stressed, but should be relatively normal, easily controlled, without much force.

Ready? Set! Go!

Control Pause (CP) - your breathing metric

What do CP numbers mean?

The length of your CP corresponds to the severity of symptoms caused by overbreathing. The greater your breathing volume, the shorter your CP will be. The longer your CP, the better oxygenated your body will be. So, when you overbreathe, your body is less able to assimilate oxygen.

When CP is 10 seconds and under:

* Asthma, sleep-related or cardio-vascular symptoms are severe;
* Breathlessness, wheezing and coughing will be frequently present both day and night;
* You may also experience several other symptoms such as rhinitis, phlegm build up, headaches, sleeplessness, lethargy and difficulty concentrating;
* Relative breathing volume is very high.

When CP is less than 20 seconds:

* Coughing, wheezing, breathlessness, exercise-induced asthma, snoring are often present;
* Tiredness, headaches, susceptibility to cough and mucus in the upper and lower respiratory systems are likely.

When CP is between 20 and 40 seconds:

* The main symptoms, as described above, are greatly reduced or disappear completely;
* Your breathing will be a lot calmer, You should not experience any night episodes of apnoea or sport-induced asthma;
* Likelihood of catching colds and chest infections is much lower.

When CP is more than 40 seconds:

* No symptoms should be present;
* You will be more energetic, healthy and clear-minded with easy breathing;
* To ensure a permanent physiological change, it is necessary to attain a morning CP of 40 seconds for at least six months.

What to expect with your CP measurements:

- Your CP should increase by at least 3-4 seconds per week during the first couple of weeks of your breathing program (doing reduced-volume breathing exercises daily);
- Physical exercise can be gradually introduced to increase your CP above 20 seconds;
- You will feel better each time your CP increases by 5 seconds;

- You can also take you CP throughout the day to provide feedback of your symptoms at different time or to identify triggers;
- Your goal is to achieve morning CP of 40 seconds for at least six months;
- Set yourself a goal for the next six months, be realistic, apply grit and get the results you deserve to live a healthier, happier life.

TIPS TO INCREASE YOUR CONTROL PAUSE

Stop breathing big

- Close your mouth and breathe through the nose day and night;
- Stop sighing. If you feel a sigh coming, try to swallow it or hold your breath;
- Apply gentle, calm, quiet breathing at all times;
- Yawn with your mouth closed.

Practise RVB (reduced-volume breathing)

Use the exercises in this program to reduce breathing volume and improve your symptoms. Each exercise has its own purpose and can be practised daily with minimal changes to your routine.

Practise physical exercise with correct breathing

Physical exercise is necessary to increase the CP from 20 to 40 seconds. Breathe through your nose as much as possible and try to keep your breathing calm and regular while you exercise. You should only need to open your mouth to breathe when performing high-intensity exercise, which is not advisable for anyone with a CP below 20 seconds.

Breathing Exercises - change your blood chemistry

Think of the following exercises as a gym for your brain. It will take time for the receptors in the respiratory centre of your brain to change their ways, their modus operandi. It is normal to experience slight discomfort when you do the exercises outlined below. The more you practice, the easier it will get.

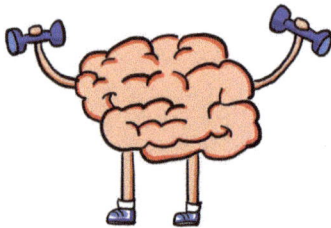

Exercise 1. Decongestant exercise

This is your unmedicated nasal drops. Use this exercise before doing any breathwork, or any physical exercises, to be able to breathe through the nose. The decongestant exercise is fantastic for those who are prone to sinus issues and find themselves slightly congested in the morning.

In all exercises, below, whenever a breath hold is required, it is done after exhalation, on "empty" lungs.

How to:

1. Breathe in, out, pinch your nose and rock your head gently up and down;
2. Keep holding your breath and rocking your head until you absolutely can't hold your breath any longer, but not to the point of dizziness;
3. Upon releasing the nose, resume breathing through the nose (mouth CLOSED at all times). The first breath in will be a big gasp (through the nose) and that's normal;
4. Once you recover your normal breathing pattern, repeat steps 1-4 three-five times.

Exercise 2. Reduced-volume breathing (RVB)

In the Oxygen Revolution Functional Breathing program this is a basic, medium intensity breath-holding exercise for breathing retraining. With the help of "reduced-volume breathing" exercise we retrain the receptors in the respiratory centre of the brain to adapt to healthier, more functional levels of carbon dioxide in the blood. It is carbon dioxide that drives your respiration, not oxygen, so befriending CO2 is the way to go!

Carbon dioxide helps oxygen detach from the hemoglobin molecule and get into the cells. Imagine a hemoglobin molecule as a taxi and CO2 as a helpful guy, who opens the door for oxygen, to get out of the taxi.

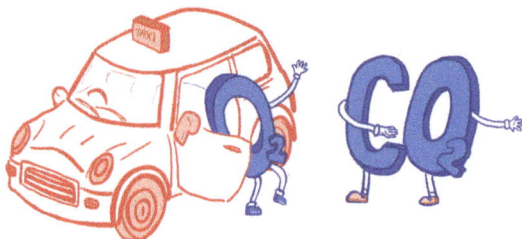

How to:

1. Sit up straight;
2. Put your index finger under the nose, like a moustache, and notice the amount of air flowing through in and out of your nostrils;

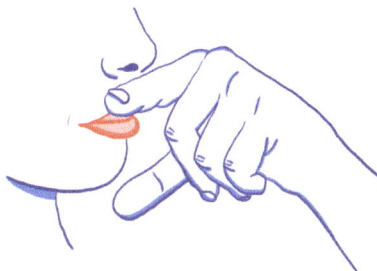

3. Gently breathe into the tip of your nostrils taking in just enough air to fill your nostrils and no more. Breathe in a flicker of air with each breath;
4. To help you reduce the amount of air you breathe in and out, these visuals may be useful: as you exhale, pretend that your finger is a feather, breathing out so gently that the feather fibres do not flutter; or imagine breathing 1cm of air in and out;
5. The temperature of the exhaled air correlates to the volume of your breathing. The warmer the air, the bigger the breath. Concentrate on slowing down your breathing to reduce the amount of warm air you feel on your finger. As you reduce and slow your

breathing you will begin to feel a mild need for air;

6. Try to maintain this need for air ("air hunger") for about 3 minutes. The air hunger should be noticeable without being stressful – the same feeling of breathlessness you might experience during a light walk. If your need for air is not distinct then gently reduce your breathing further. If your need for air is too stressful, then allow your body to relax and take in a little more air with each breath;

7. I recommend you put a timer on your phone for 4 minutes and relax into the process until you hear the timer going off. Repeat the exercise 3-4 times with one-minute break between the rounds. It is important to recover your breath between reps;

8. The need for air during this exercise should be tolerable, not stressful at all;

9. Remember, that you are in control of your breathing at all times. Experiment. Approach this exercise with curiosity – what is your body capable of? How does it function? What is your tolerance to CO_2? How can you improve it and help your magnificent body, using the power of your mind and determination to get better?

This exercise is to be done twice a day (more if time allows).

Exercise 3. Steps

This is a medium-to-strong intensity breath-holding exercise.

How to:

1. Take a small breath in and let a small breath out through your nose;
2. Hold your breath by pinching your nose or closing the muscles of your throat;
3. Walk as many steps as you can while maintaining the breath hold until you feel a medium to strong need for air;
4. Try to build up a large air shortage by doing as many steps as possible without losing control of your breathing;
5. Resume calm nasal breathing. (first breath in is going to be a gasp, but your goal is to calm down your breathing by the end of a one-minute break between rounds);
6. You should be able to recover from "Steps" within 10 breaths. If you cannot, you have held your breath for too long.

Count your paces during the "Steps" exercise and compare your score each day to measure your progress.

GOAL: to increase your score by 5-10 paces a week.

There is a correlation between your Control Pause (CP)

measurement and the number of paces in STEPS you can make. The higher the CP, the better the score in STEPS.

I highly recommend you start a journal to record your progress. It is super helpful if you jot down your observations of how you feel on that day, what new foods you included, any events of the day, etc. There is a significant link between your mental and emotional states and breathing (as mentioned in Chapter 1 – it is all about your nervous system!).

Notes to Steps exercise

- While you experience a strong air shortage when holding your breath and walking at the same time, it should not be stressful.
- Like all breathing exercises STEPS should be practised on an empty stomach (wait for at least 40 minutes after eating if this is the time you have).
- For first few weeks aim to do 18 repetitions of STEPS (e.g. 6-10 repetitions done 2-3 times daily).

Exercise 4. Small breath holds

In the Oxygen Revolution Functional Breathing Program we call this exercise a "breathing ventolin" for its ability to open up airways quite effectively.

This exercise is suitable for everybody – from the young to the elderly, as it is a light-intensity breath-holding exercise. It can be practised as many times a day as desired or needed. Anyone with severe asthma or emphysema should aim to practise this exercise throughout the day and into the night. It is gentle, safe and will dramatically reduce the symptoms.

How to:

1. Sit down comfortably;
2. Breathe in, out, pinch your nose and hold your breath for 5 seconds (or 5 counts);
3. Release the breath hold, keep breathing through the nose, mouth is CLOSED at all times, for 10 seconds;
4. Repeat for 3-5 minutes.

Breathing exercises - improve breathing mechanics

This part is overlooked or not taught properly in many available breath courses. However you cannot leave the mechanics of breathing without attention.

Exercise 1. 360° breathing

360-degree breathing is exactly what is in the name. Have you ever noticed an animal breathe? Observe your dog or cat – they don't breathe with their tummy, their whole rib cage expands! This is how we, humans, are designed to breathe as well.

How to:

1. Lie down comfortably on a firm surface – a yoga mat, carpet, rug;
2. Put your hands on the sides of the lower ribs and feel them expanding, pushing into your hands when you breathe in, and imagine your waist going small and ribs coming close together when you breathe out (squeezing all the air out gently, without force);
3. Next step here is to feel your spine pushing into the mat as you breathe in, creating the 360° breathing technique - the ribcage expands all around;
4. Do this exercise while maintaining slow gentle nasal breathing - breathe in to the count of 4, breathe out to the count of 6.

Exercise 2. Opening the back

360-degree breathing is what we aim for here as well as in the previous exercise. Even your back opens up ever so slightly. This is a stretching exercise which can be performed while sitting down and standing. It helps open up your back and achieve that all-around breathing pattern. The movement is the least in the back when we breathe, as compared to the sides, but there should be a sensation of widening. Most often tight muscles and bracing during training make back expansions next to impossible. This muscle retraining starts with awareness and tuning into the sensations in your back when breathing, feeling the back elongating on inhalation.

How to:

1. Stand/sit with your back straight (imagine a string attached to the top of your head and someone is pulling the string up, opening up your spine) with your arms stretched out in front of you, hands interlocked, palms facing outward);
2. Expand your back on the inhale, pushing into the back and resisting into the palms;
3. Back to neutral on the exhale.

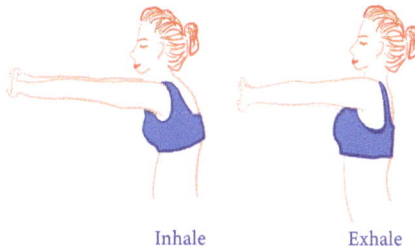

Inhale   Exhale

Exercise 3. Cat-cow stretch for 360° breathing

The mechanical theory behind this exercise is similar to Exercise 2 "Opening the back". We try to open the back on the inhale and contract, coming to neutral, on the exhale.

How to:

This exercise can be done as traditionally taught in yoga, standing on your fours, or with the help of a stable chair while standing with your legs straight, knees slightly bent.

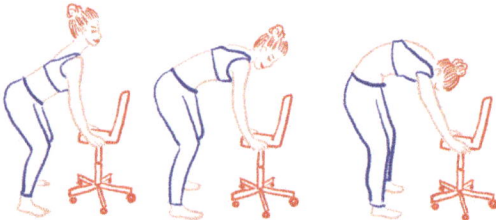

Inhale   Start exhalation   End of exhale

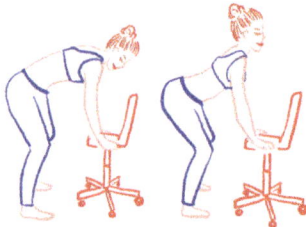

Inhale   End of inhale

Exercise 4. Child's pose

This is a back-opening exercise.

How to:

Assume the Child's pose with arms by the sides (left picture below). This is your position for breathing in. Feel your back expanding and the ribs expanding laterally.
Bring your upper body up (back straight), approximately to 45 degrees, do not sit all the way up. While you are coming up, breathe out, gently squeezing your pelvic floor muscles and engaging the core. No hard bracing!

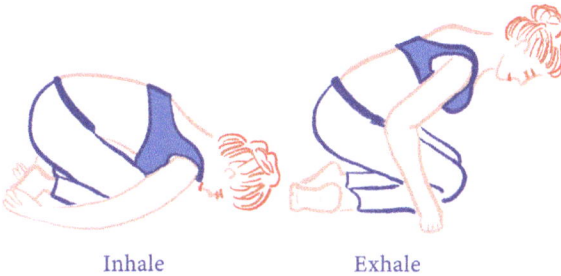

Inhale   Exhale

Exercise 5. Intercostal stretch

Intercostal muscles fall into the category of primary (main) breathing muscles. Your ability to use them will ensure optimal lung expansion and oxygenation of the tissues.

How to:

Follow the step-by-step picture instructions below.

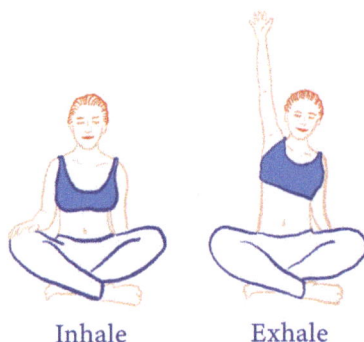

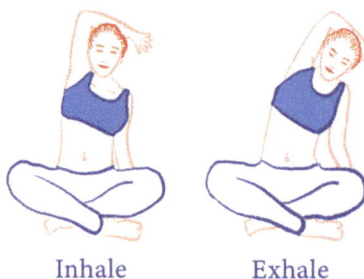

Inhale   Exhale

Inhale   Exhale

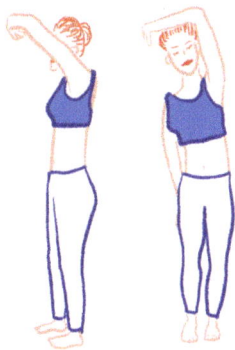

Inhale   Exhale

Variation

"Our character is basically a composite of our habits."

Stephen R. Covey

MAINTAIN

So, you have achieved some progress – your CP has gotten up, you have more stamina when working out, you don't get out of breath too fast when walking or hiking. How to maintain that level of health? Like with anything in life, adopting breathwork as part of your lifestyle is the only way to go. Now that you have the basics covered, I encourage you to experiment. Get really curious about your potential, about what is possible for the physical body you choose to inhabit. Modify the breath-holding exercises to suit your emotional and metabolic needs. What if you challenge yourself and do an X amount of rounds in the morning and notice how that affects your day? Doing breath holding after exhaling, before going into a meeting, doing public speaking, etc., is going to improve the oxygen delivery to your brain and make you more alert and energised. Use the power of breath to achieve your goals in life!

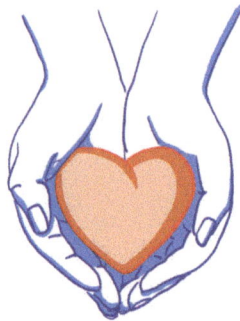

When anxious, put both hands on your heart, slow down your breath, drop into the heart space. Breathe in and out into the solar plexus, feeling the diaphragm contract and relax. After a couple of slow breaths like that, through the nose, say out loud or in your head: "I am OK, I am safe, I am loved." Because right now, in this moment, you are.

Once you get your functional breathing metrics to a decent level (think of your Control Pause measurement – refer to "Control Pause (CP) - your breathing metric" on page 32, do not limit yourself to the information in this book. This book's goal is to take your health to an optimal baseline level, from where you can build up as the foundation has been set solid and sound. Explore other types of breathwork – pranayamas, dragon breathing, holotropic breath, Wim Hof style. The only thing I recommend is to do it with the only purpose of self-discovery, to learn more about your body, its connection to your mind and emotions. Learn to take notice and observe, don't do it just for a tick.

Exercise to connect to the heart and develop your intuition

And here is a little bonus for you – an exercise to help you connect to your magnificent body even deeper, to use the breath as a medium to allow yourself to tune into your physiology. The more you are attuned to your body, the better you listen to it, the easier you navigate this life in all areas – work, relationship, etc. Your body never creates a disease, it only adapts and responds to the inputs you subject it to. And it speaks to you via sensations, aches and pains. This is the only way that your body can get your attention that some things are not good for you, some actions are out of alignment with who you are, some thoughts, which you choose to keep, may not be serving your health any longer, and it's time to reconsider.

This exercise brings your heart connection to the next level. You will gain access to the ability to sense your heart – its rate, its state. It is an advanced exercise, so don't be discouraged if it takes time to get to do it successfully.

After you have that long inhale and exhale, start seeing where in your body you can feel your pulse. Close your eyes and see if you can feel it. It could be a pulsating sensation inside your ears, a feeling in your fingers, abdomen, neck. Practice feeling your heart rate. And the level up from this is to play with the amount of noise around you - music in the background, children playing loudly, coffee machine working, etc. See if you can sense your heart rate when you are experiencing different emotions – anger, elation, frustration. Once you feel it, I challenge you to guess it (do it for roughly 10 seconds and multiply by 6 to get heart rate per minute). Use a heart rate monitor or an app on your phone to see how close you are. Change the setting to more or less loud, more or less emotional, and play the guessing game again!

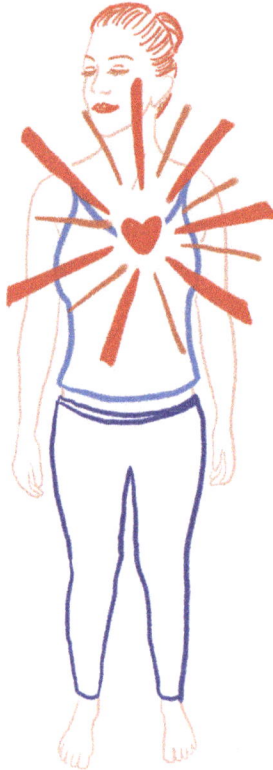

Summary of the main functional breathing concepts

This is what I'd like you to take away with you after reading this little practical functional breathing manual (and my hope is that these main concepts of functional breathing become your lifestyle):

- Nasal breathing is essential for good health, longevity and energy;
- Breathing mechanics matter: by using your diaphragm you not only open up the lower lobes of the lungs, providing more oxygen to the body, but you also massage the abdominal organs, helping digestion; diaphragmatic breathing also helps you detoxify by moving the lymph better. And lastly, diaphragmatic breathing helps the vagal tone;
- "Breathe, as if you are not breathing" - gentle, inaudible breath is what you are aiming for;
- The slower your breathing rate is, the better off your overall health is. Four-to-six ratio is the gold standard in functional breathing.

INSPIRATION

I had to finish the book with this chapter. I would love you to get inspired by your respiration. Both words – "inspiration" and "respiration" have the word "spirit" as a root. Respiration is our link with something bigger than us. We inhale the matter of the universe and exhale, blending our existence with the eternal, endless world we are part of. If you think about it for a moment, it is pretty damned breathtaking (pun intended).

This chapter is my favourite as we all need reminders about the infinite, the important, the WHY. Personally, I refer to the quotes from this chapter quite often myself, they keep me accountable (to myself) and serve as a prompt to go back to the basics when life challenges seem overwhelming.

Inspiration in life, at times, must be lovingly nurtured by us. We literally breathe life into projects, ideas, actions, by breathing well into our physical bodies. Inspiration, our drive, motivation are closely linked to this essential function which our body performs for us - respiration. We don't even think about it, our breathing is automatic. And the beauty of it is that if it gets out of balance, we can direct it. We can harmonise our breath to restore the homeostasis in our physiology, the balance in our emotional and mental nature. We are the creators. It takes practice and I believe everyone is capable of doing it. I believe in every one of you.

I hope you enjoy these bits of inspiration.

And if no one said it to you today – you are OK, you are appreciated and you are loved.

"When you own your breath, nobody can steal your peace."

Unknown

"The most healing breathing exercise is laughter."

Nick Health

"Breath is the bridge which connects life to consciousness, which unites your body to your thoughts."

Thich Nhay Hanh

"Deep breaths are like little love notes to your body."

Unknown

"Breathe. Let go. And remind yourself that this very moment is the only one you know you have for sure."

Oprah Winfrey

"The better you think of yourself, the better your chances of being well."

Dr. Robert Fulford

"Six months from now, you're going to look back at your life and say 'I really did believe in myself' and it worked!"

Unknown

"The gap between where you want to be and where you are right now comes down to your habits, discipline and mindset."

Unknown

"Simplicity is difficult to implement in modern life because it is against the spirit of certain brand of people who seek sophistication so they can justify their profession."

Taleb

"Breathing is an effective, free and simple remedy for multiple ailments. It's hard to believe that something that simple can be that powerful."

Julia Rudakova

"If something is humanly possible, it's attainable by you too."

Marcus Aurelius

"It's not about feeling better, it's about getting better at feeling."

Gabor Maté

"Feelings come and go like clouds in a windy sky. Conscious breathing is my anchor."

Unknown

"Live a life where you wouldn't even need or be interested in learning about 'how to heal'."

Dr. Huckaby

"Your mind will answer most questions if you learn to relax and wait for the answer."

William Burroghs

"Sometimes the most important thing in a whole day is the rest we take between two deep breaths."

Etty Hillesum

"From our first breath to our last, awe moves us to deepen our relations with the wonders of life and to marvel at the vast mysteries that are part of our fleeting time here, guided by this most human of emotions."

Dacher Keltner

"Breathe deeply, until sweet air extinguishes the burn of fear in your lungs and every breath is a beautiful refusal to become anything less than infinite."

D. Antoinette Foy

"Deep breathing brings deep thinking and shallow breathing brings shallow thinking."

Elsie Lincoln Benedict

"When the breath is unsteady, all is unsteady; when the breath is still; all is still. Control the breath carefully. Inhalation gives strength and a controlled body; retention gives steadiness of mind and longevity; exhalation purifies body and spirit."

Goraksasatakam

"If you woke up breathing, congratulations! You have another chance."

Andrea Boydston

"Inhale, then exhale. That's how you'll get through it."

Unknown

"What has to be taught first is the breath."

Confucious

"The secret of life is right under your nose!"

Dan Brule

"Breathing control gives man strength, vitality, inspiration, and magic powers."

Zhuangzi

"I love to breathe. Oxygen is sexy!"

Kris Carr

"Focusing on the act of breathing clears the mind of all daily distractions and clears our energy enabling us to better connect with the Spirit within."

Unknown

"Remember, as long as you are breathing it's never too late to start a new beginning."

Unknown

"Regulate the breathing, and thereby control the mind."

B.K.S. Iyengar

"Let go of the battle. Breathe quietly and let it be. Let your body relax and your heart soften."

Jack Komfield

"When you practice mindfulness of breathing, then the breathing is mind."

Thich Nhat Hanh

"In today's busy world it is essential to take a moment to breathe and cultivate mindfulness at work."

Unknown

"The best way to predict the future is to create it, and mindfulness helps us stay focused on the present moment to make the most of our life."

Unknown

"Breathing in, I am aware that I am breathing in.
Breathing out, I am aware that I am breathing out.
Breathing in, I am grateful for this moment.
Breathing out, I smile.
Breathing in, I am aware of the preciousness of this day.
Breathing out, I vow to live deeply in this day."

Thich Nhat Hanh

ABOUT THE AUTHOR

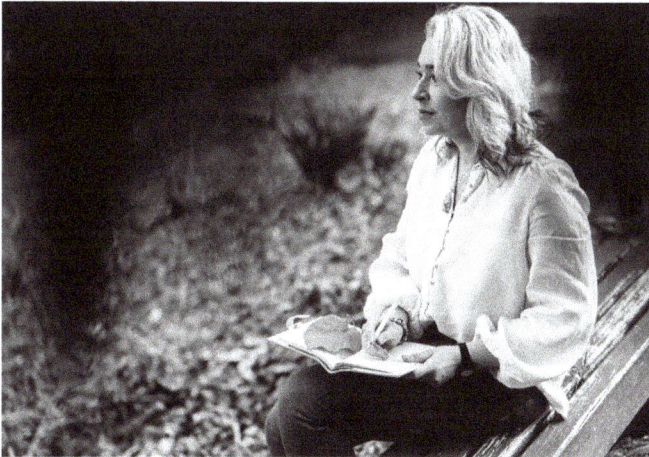

Julia Rudakova is a naturopath who specialises in respiratory conditions and has been running the Oxygen Revolution functional breathing program for adults and children online and at her clinic in Melbourne, Australia. Her passion to use breathwork as the first step to healing stems from her personal health journey as well as her extensive research into respiratory health and in the link between breathing and mental and emotional health.

Julia has a gift of distilling complex concepts into simple, actionable pieces of information, and this book is the result of her applied skill to do exactly that. Her mission is to help individuals take charge of their health, feel empowered and savour the life they're given.

Learn more at: *https://www.oxygenrevolution.com.au/*

FROM THE SAME AUTHOR

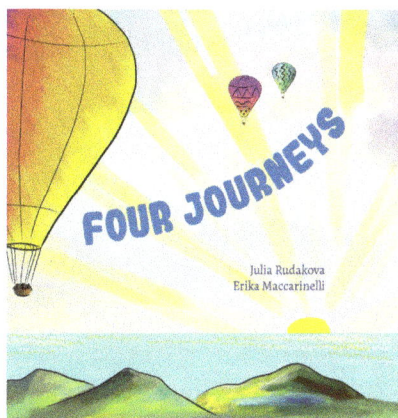

Beautifully illustrated, **Four Journeys** is a book for families who want to achieve the best of health. The journeys along four different landscapes take you through four interactive breathing exercises. The use of bright images to keep a child's attention, and the engagement of kinaesthetic learning will help bring focus to breathing and re-educate the brain and body to breathe in a health-conducive way.

The benefits of doing the breathing exercises include reduced incidents of ear-nose-throat diseases, well-balanced nervous system and proper craniofacial development. All of this leads to reduced anxiety and behavioural problems, improved sleep, beautiful smiles and overall calmness.

Only 5 minutes of fun practice twice a day can set you and your family on the path of a joyful journey to health.

https://www.oxygenrevolution.com.au/four-journeys